Daylight

A True Story of Childhood Schizophrenia

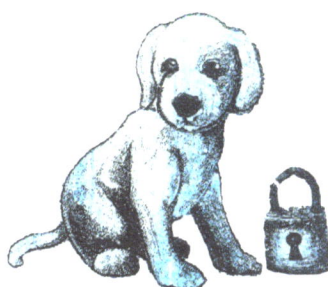

By Daniel-James F. Clarke and Cynthia Kaufman-Rose
Illustrated by Cynthia Kaufman-Rose

SUNNY DAY®
PUBLISHING, LLC

Daylight
A True Story of Childhood Schizophrenia

Printed in the United States of America

Sunny Day Publishing, LLC
www.sunnydaypublishing.com

ISBN 978-0-9825480-9-7

Dedication

For Todd Ivan, MD and Dr. Robert Byrnes, my true friends.
For my mother, Mary Jo Clarke, one in a million.
And for Axil, who was more than just a dog.

— Daniel

With love for my children, Emma, Asher and Clara, and for my husband, Kyle.
In honor of my parents, Inge and Jozsi, hidden children of the Shoah.
And for Evy. May insight unlock your dreams.

— Cynthia

Daniel always sleeps with the lights on.
So does his dog, Axil.

Dreams seem less real this way.

In the nighttime, while he's asleep, Daniel dreams.
He dreams a piano is playing music.

He dreams about red bicycles, shining stars,
and book pages turning.

Axil dreams about biscuits.

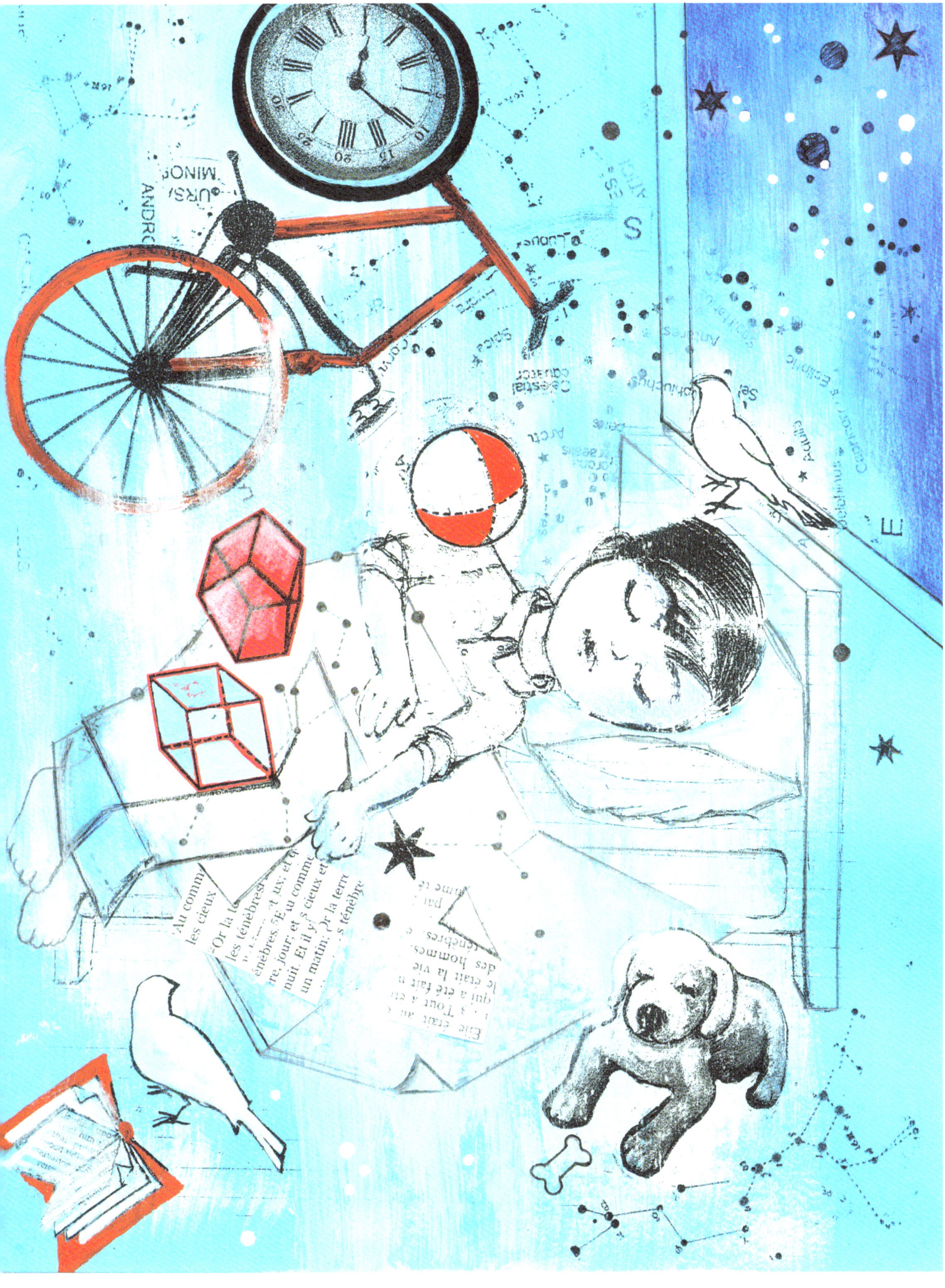

In the daylight, while he's awake, Daniel dreams.

He dreams about glass prisms and opening boxes.
He hears stars whisper and birds telling secrets.
It seems like everything is whispering.

Sometimes the daydreams are real.
Sometimes they aren't.

Daniel doesn't know the difference.

He can't tell if the things he sees and hears are real
or daydreams.

Everything seems like a daydream to Daniel.

Except for Axil.
Daniel knows Axil is real.

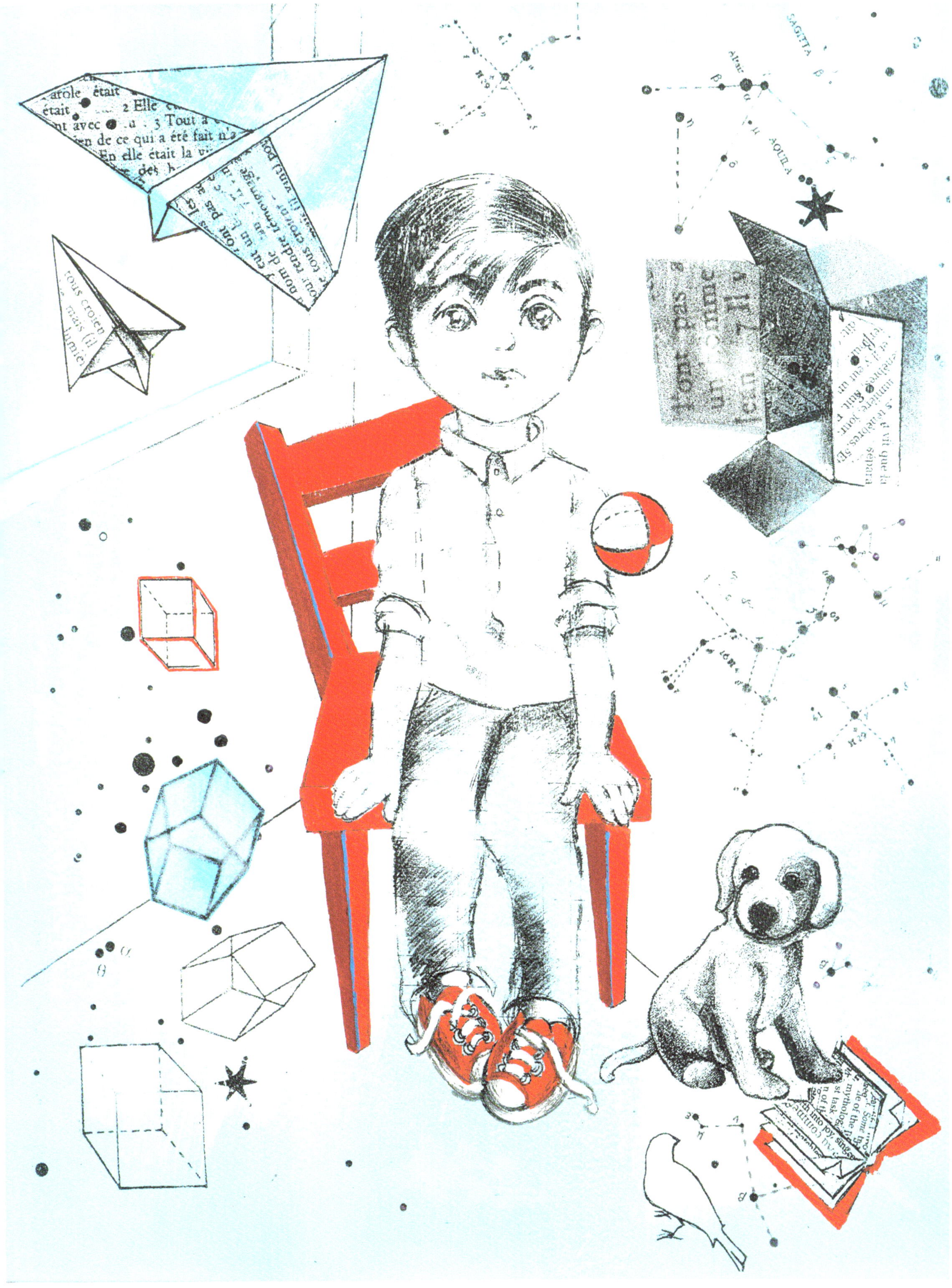

At breakfast, Daniel daydreams about wet umbrellas dripping
and paper airplanes whistling.
He smells salty rainwater.
He hears paper folding.

Some of the daydreams Daniel can see and hear.
And some of the daydreams he can touch, smell and taste.

Sometimes paper airplanes and breakfast taste the same.

Axil likes to taste everything.

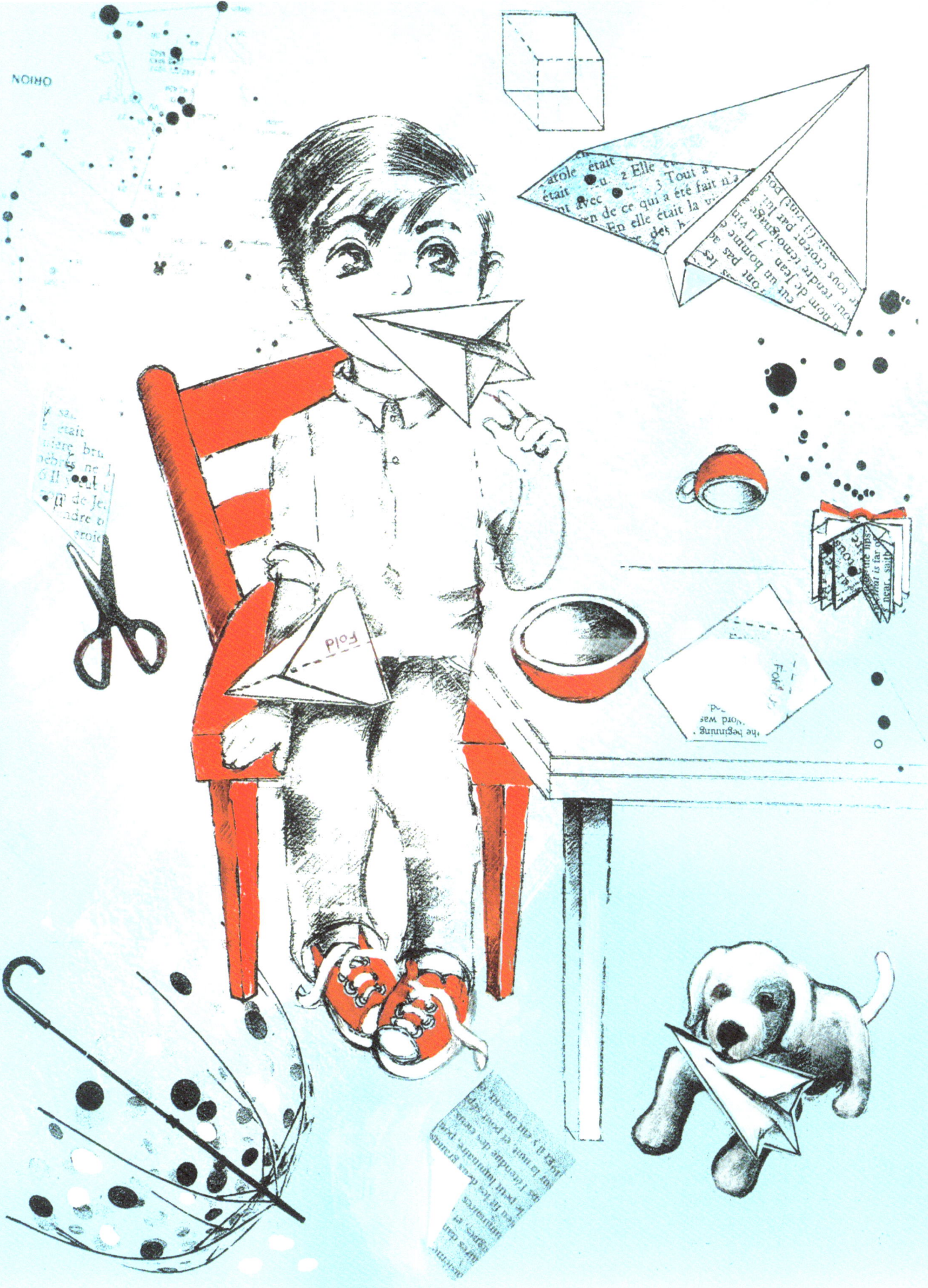

A clock ticks on the wall at school.

The teacher doesn't notice a bird on her head.

Daniel notices.
If Axil were allowed in school, he would notice.
But no one else notices.

Birds peck on the teacher's desk.
No one else hears the birds.

Letters on the chalkboard laugh.
No one else hears the letters.

Except for Daniel.
He hears everything.

He starts to laugh.
He tries to stay quiet, but laughs even louder.

Then Daniel hears a paper bag tear in two.

The teacher looks down.
An empty bag is on the floor.

"What happened to my lunch?" she asks.

Daniel sees a tail wag under her desk.

This time, the class starts to giggle.
But this time Daniel stays quiet.

Peanut butter is Axil's favorite.

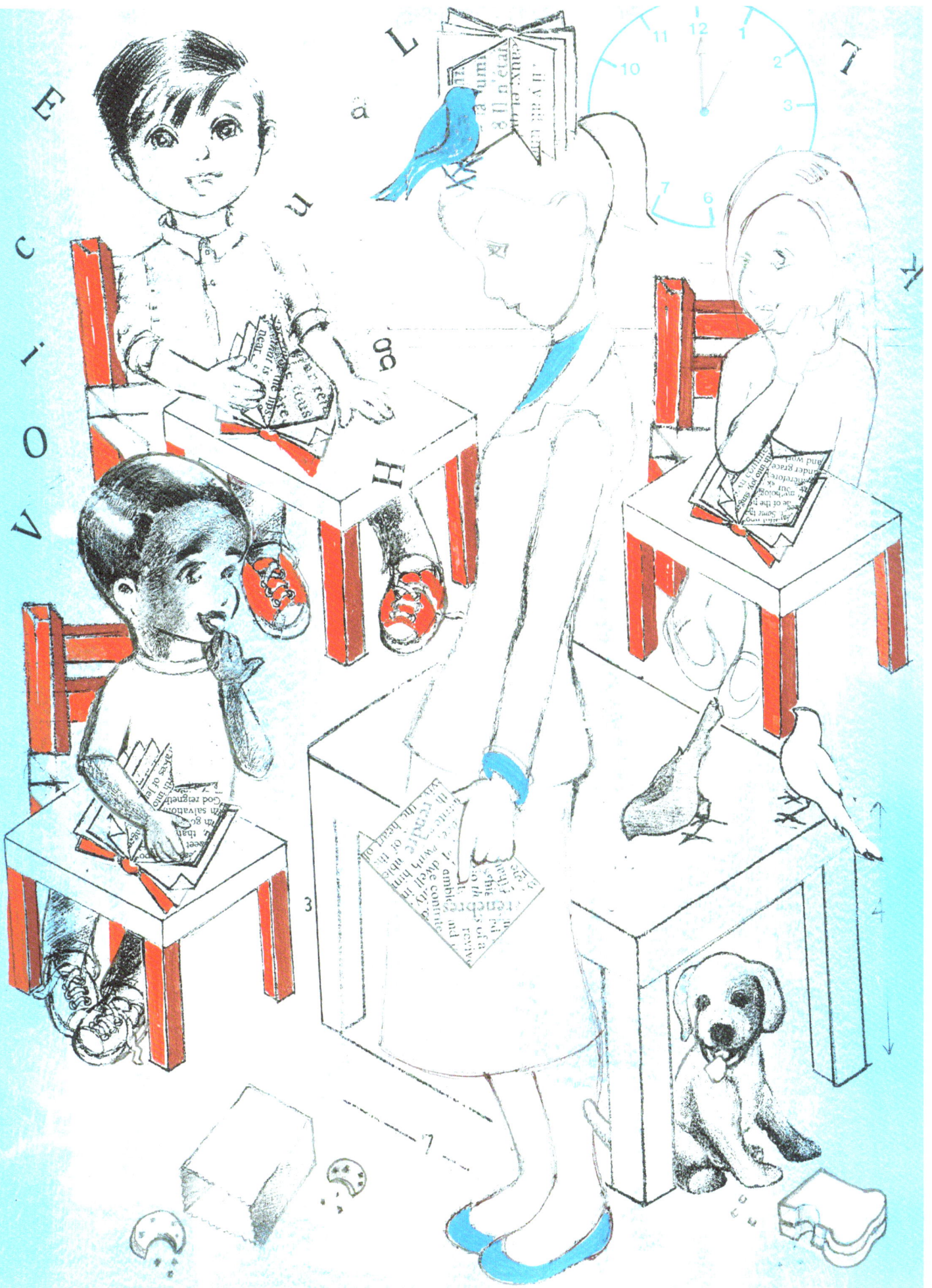

Sometimes everything is moving.
Other times everything stays still.
Sometimes everything is upside-down.

Axil is always right side up.

Daniel hears letters talking about him.
He hears teachers whispering about him.
He hears kids telling what he's thinking.

He hears people on the sidewalk saying his name.

And sometimes he hears voices when nobody is there at all.

Daniel tries to laugh at the voices to make them go away.

Axil chases them.

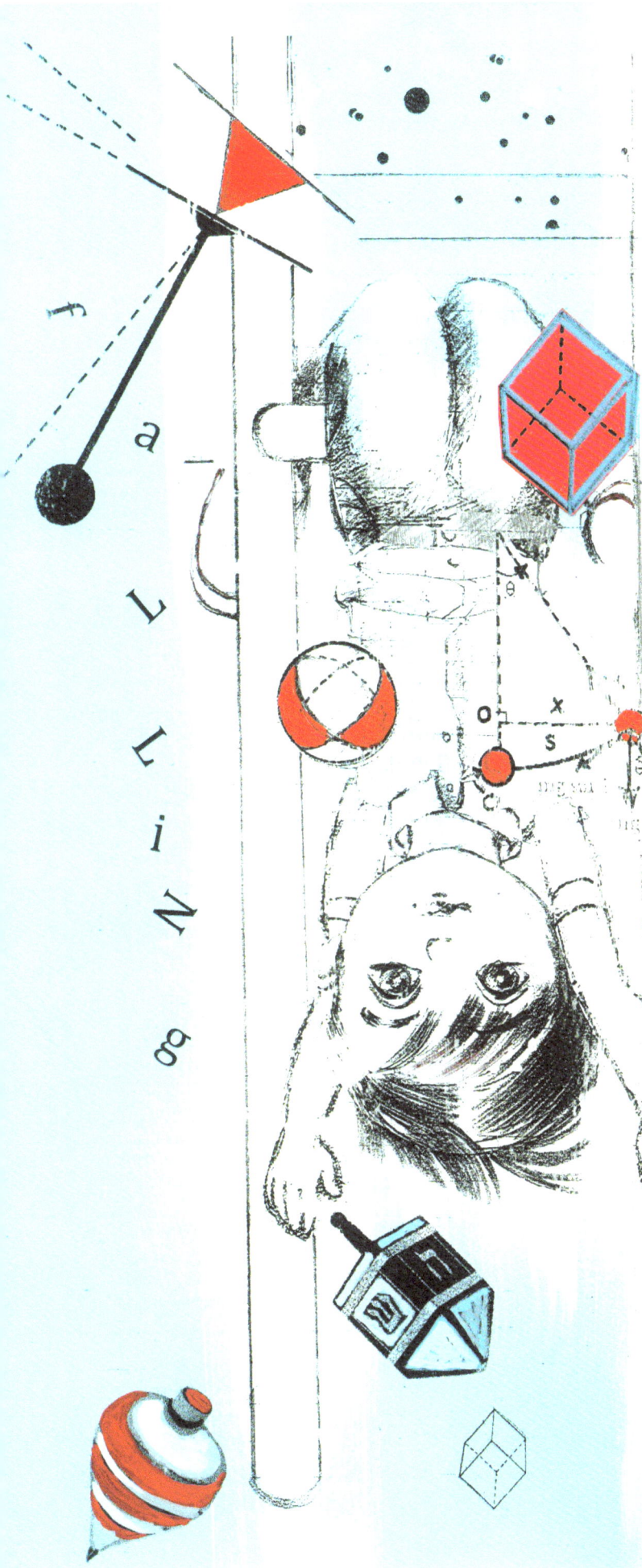

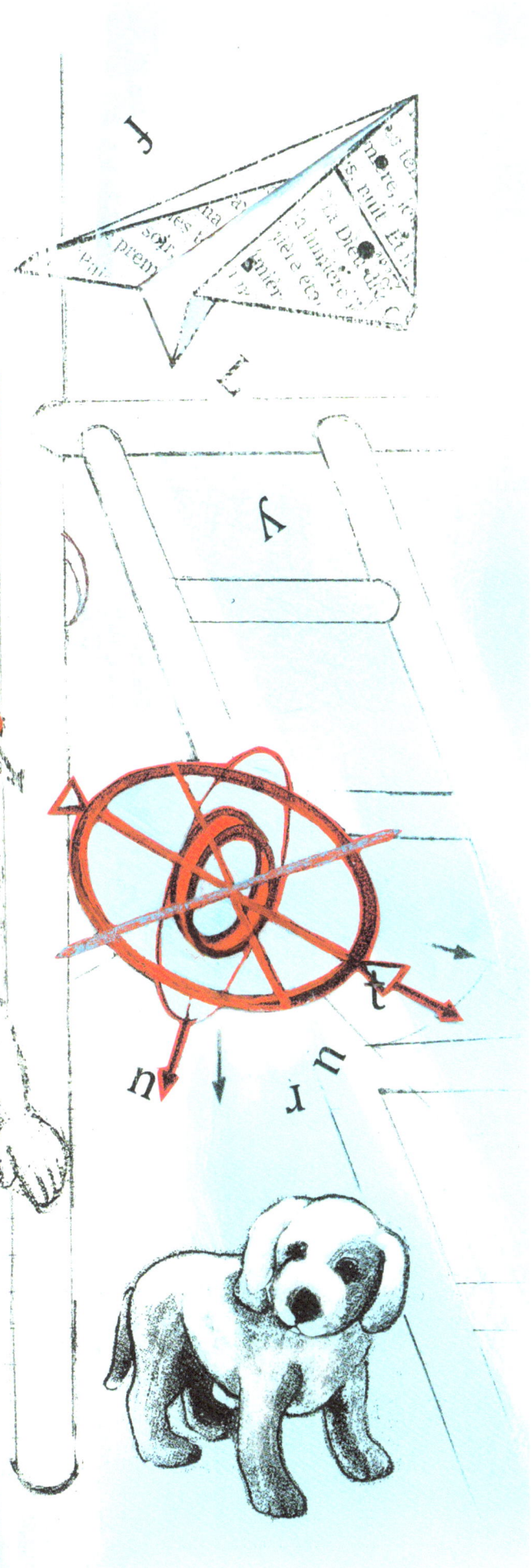

Klunk.

A shoe falls from the top of the fire escape stairs.
A boy looks up.
"How did you get up there?"

"The invisible voice told me how," Daniel replies.
"What invisible voice?"
"The one that's always telling me what to do."

"What else does it tell you?"
"Whatever it wants to."
"Is it talking now?"

"Sure," says Daniel, "it's saying watch out for the piano."
"What piano?"
"The one falling under the stairs."

"You're crazy," the boy scowls and rolls his eyes.

Axil bangs the piano keys.

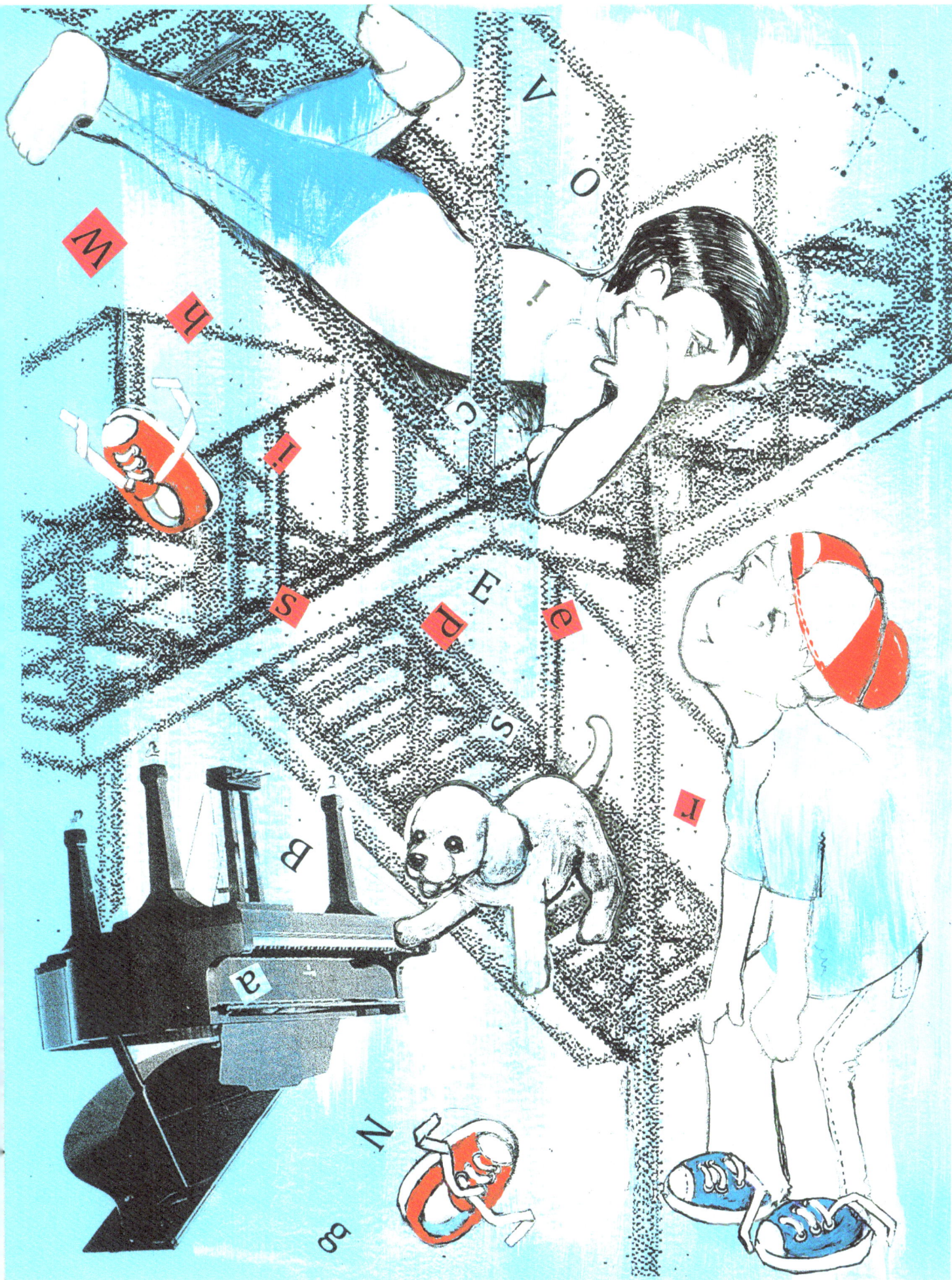

Some days the daydreams are so close and so loud,
Daniel can't see or hear real things.

Tumbling letters and numbers and boxes often cause him to trip
and fall. He walks in a strange way to avoid them.

Sometimes Daniel wanders off because he hears voices
tell him to run and catch the daydreams.
He pays more attention to the daydreams
than he does to other kids.
They can't see and hear what Daniel does, so they laugh.

The noisy laughter makes it hard for Daniel to concentrate.
It makes him ache inside.

Axil growls at the boxes.

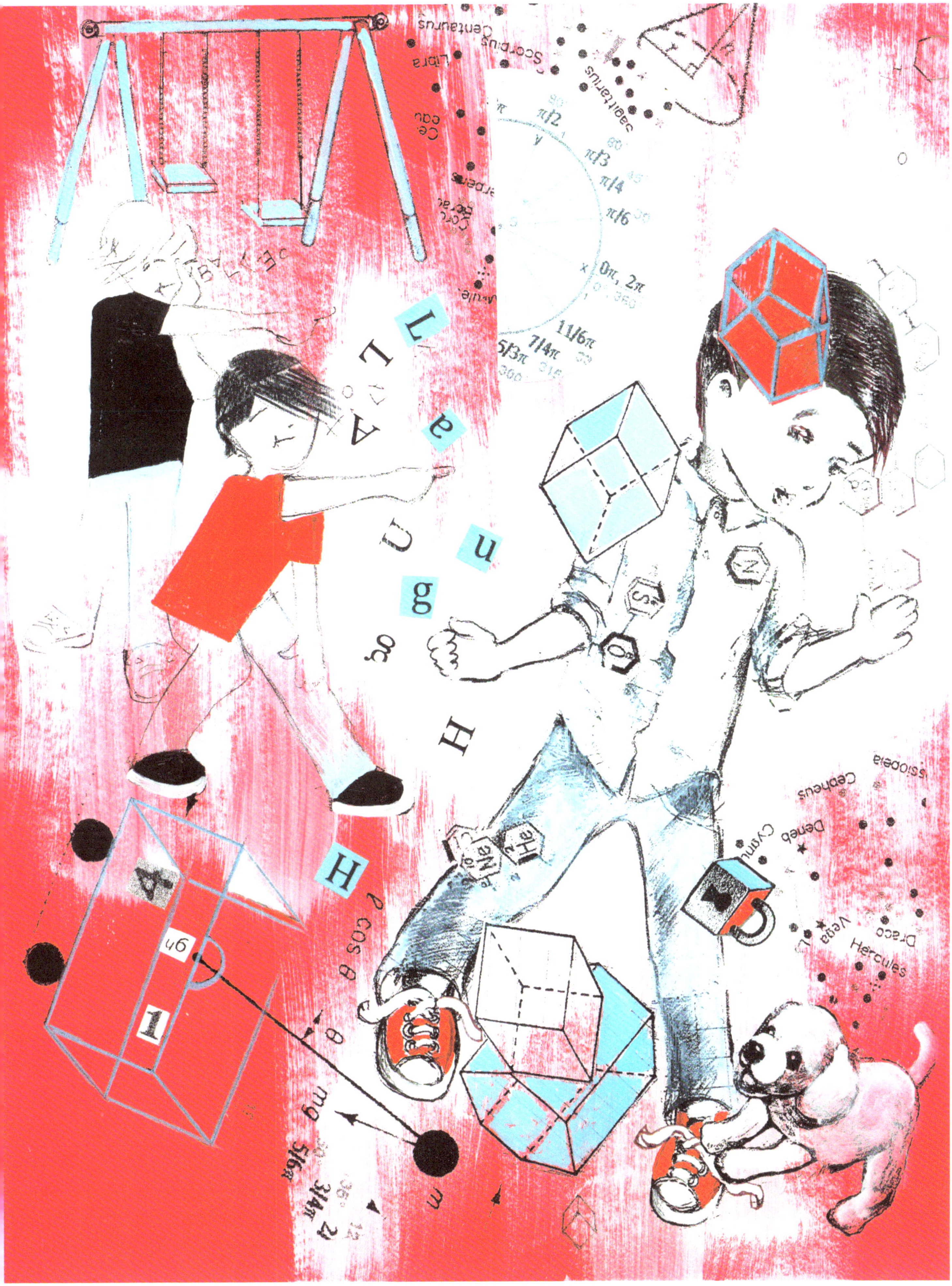

π/2
π/3
π/4
π/6
0π, 2π
11/6π
7/4π
5/3π
Scorpius
Centaurus
Libra
Sagittarius
Cepheus
Deneb
Vega
Draco
Hercules

Daniel doesn't like to be near many people.
They stare at him in a strange way.
They talk about him in a strange way.

People and voices and daydreams all together feel too crowded.
He just wants to be alone.

Alone, with Axil.

Because some of the voices and daydreams come and go quickly,
but most of them never go away.
Daniel tries to hide from them.

Axil tries to chase them away.

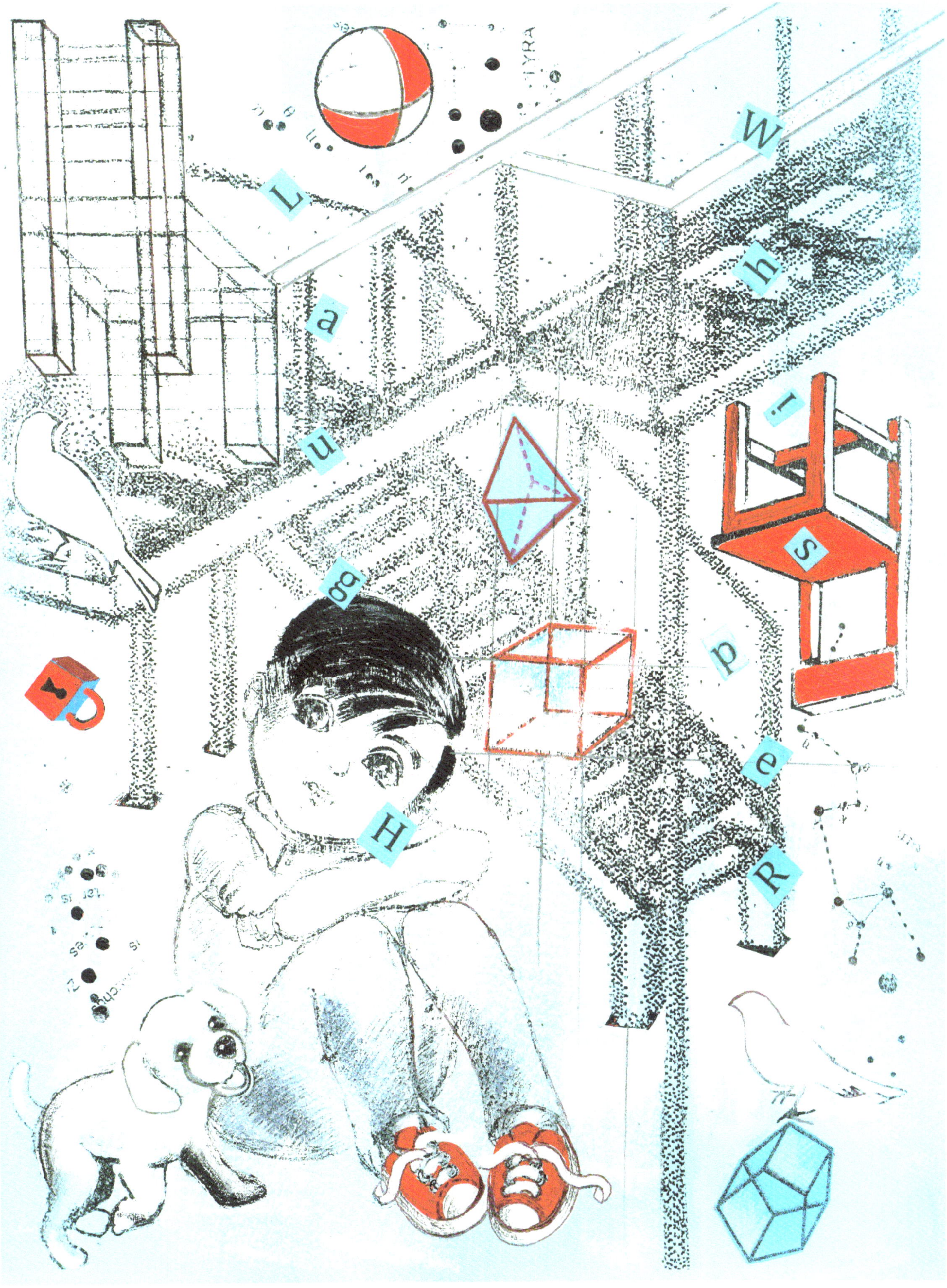
L
a
u
g
H
W
h
i
s
p
e
R
LYRA

Sometimes the daydreams are exceptionally
noisy and crowded.

The chess pieces rattle.
The book pages tear off. The letters fly up.
The bicycle screeches. The game board bangs.

Axil tries to hold everything still.
Then the wall clatters down.

Daniel hears quiet voices murmuring about him.
He hears angry voices shouting at him.
He thinks everyone is annoyed with him.

Everything is too fast and too loud.

He covers his ears.

He wishes everything would stop.

But no matter how hard Daniel tries,
he can't stop the daydreams.

And no matter how hard Axil tries, he can't catch them all.

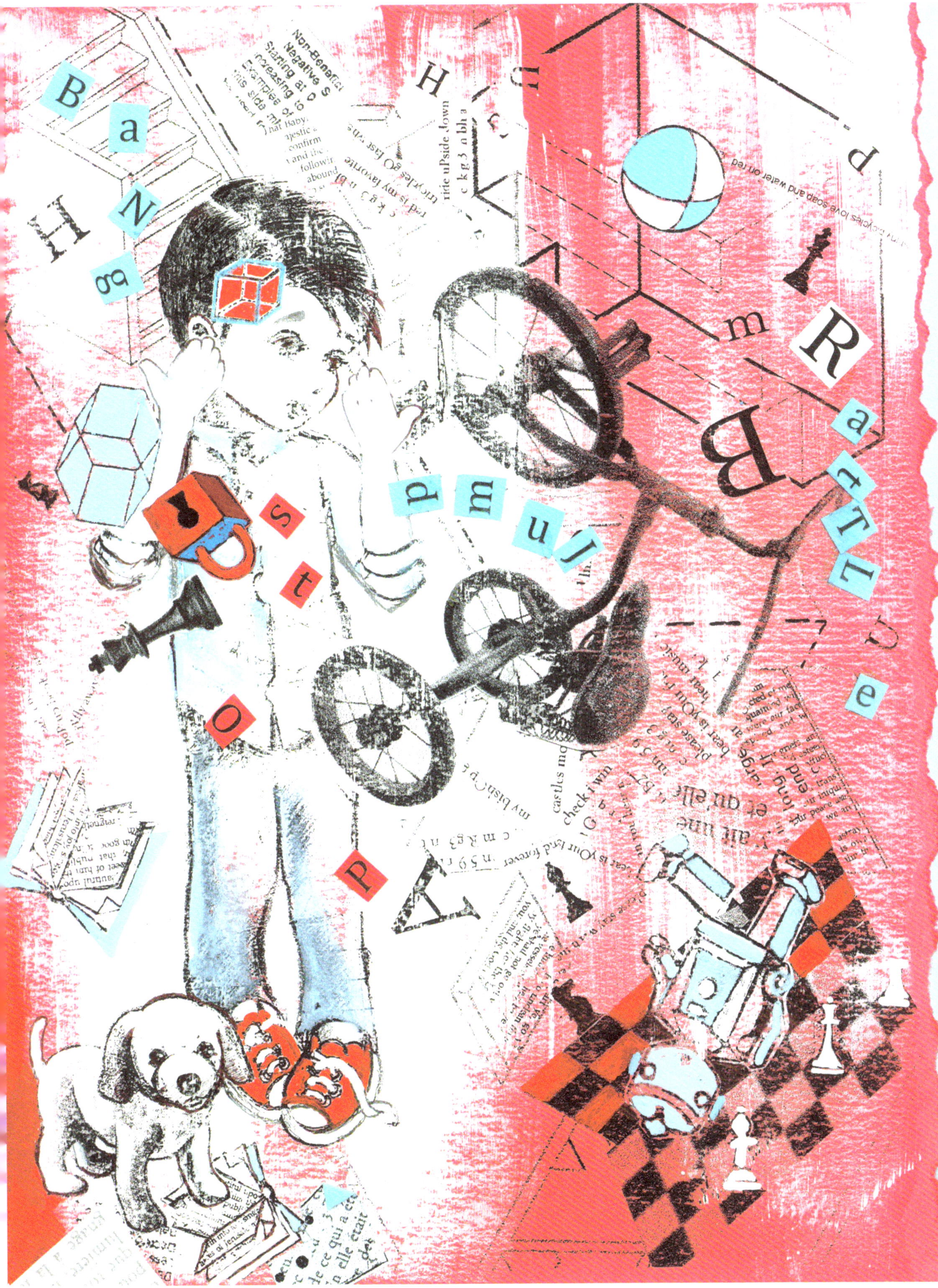
BaNg
Jump
stop
RattLe

Daniel hears a voice telling him to go outside.
He wanders out, trying not to step on the daydreams.

He runs toward the street.
The voices are so loud he can't hear the sound of the rushing cars.
Axil hears the cars, and pulls hard on Daniel's shoe.

Daniel hears his mother calling, so he goes back inside.

Axil follows close behind.

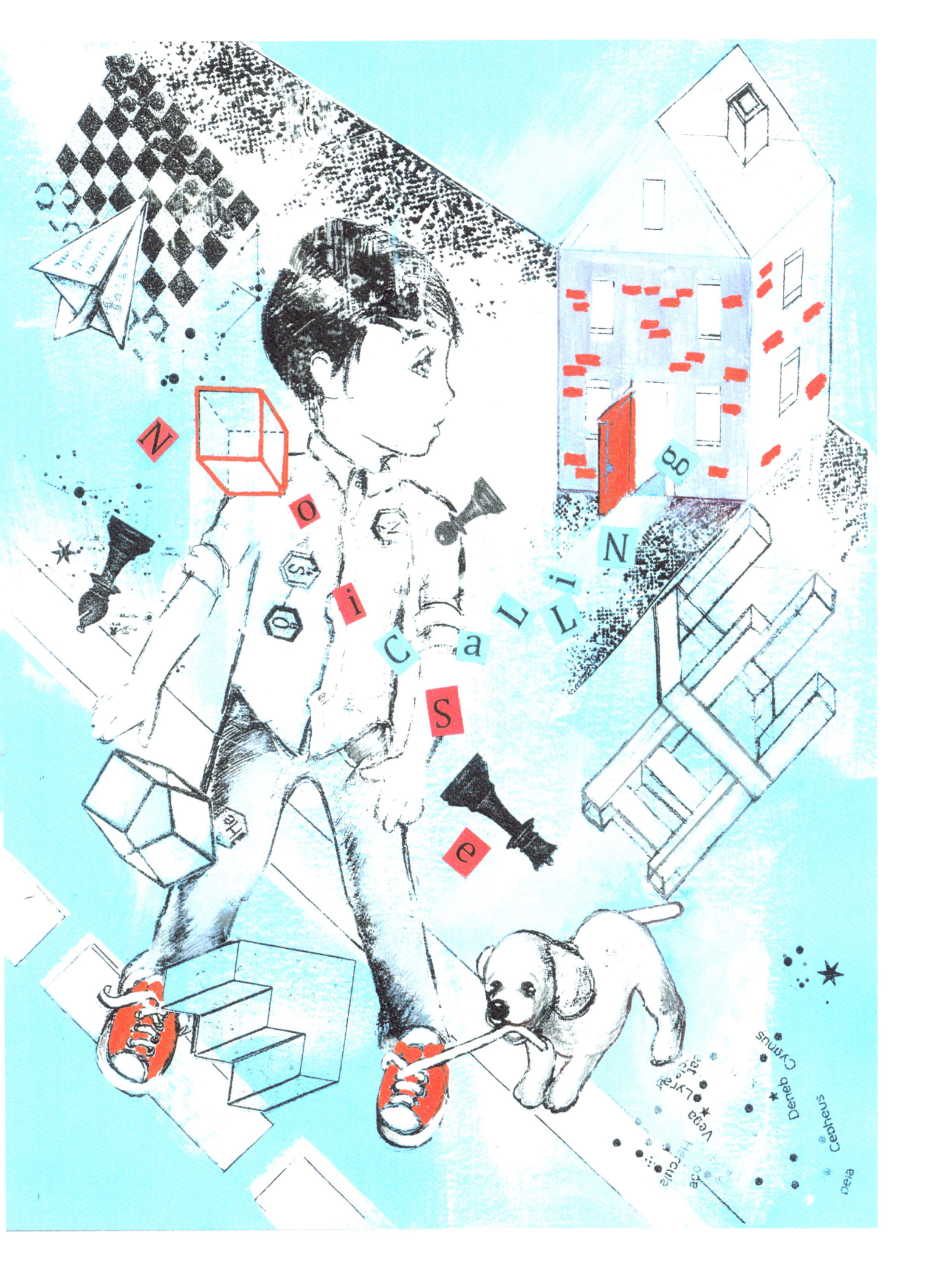

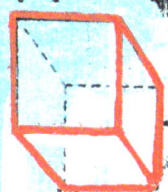

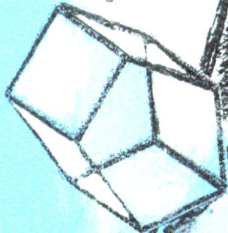

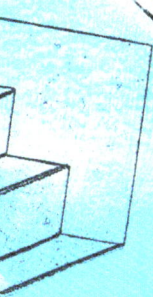

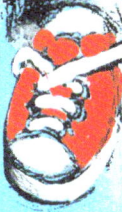

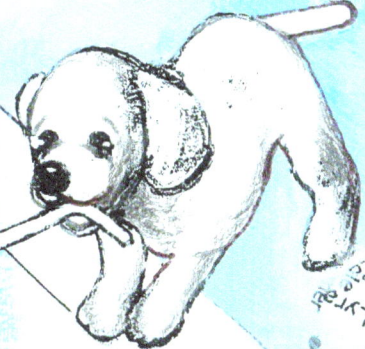

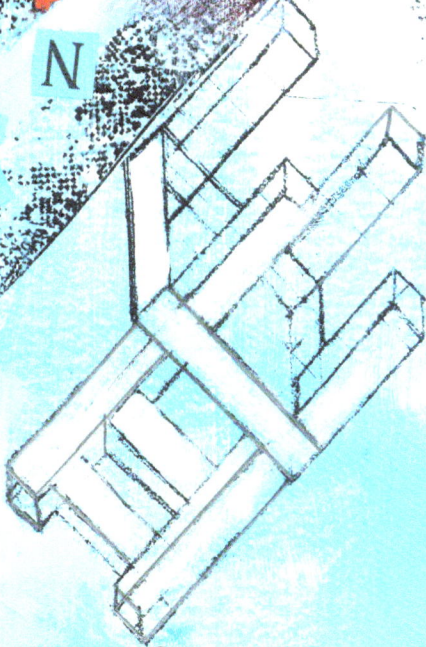

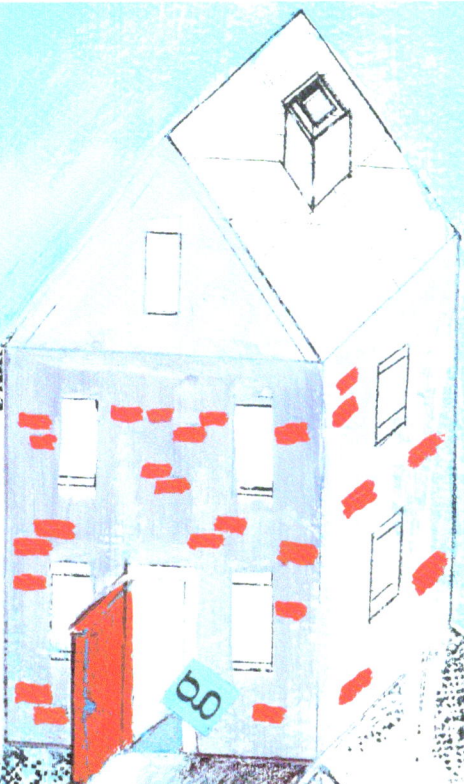

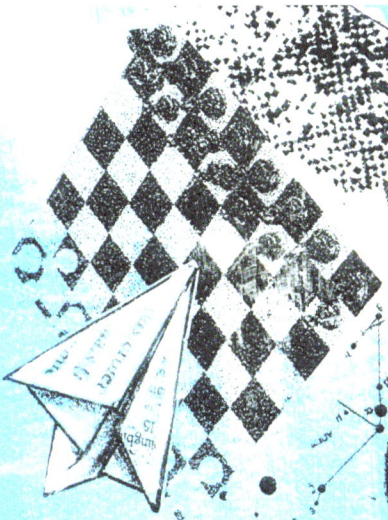

"Why are you shouting?" Daniel asks his mother.

"I didn't shout," she replies.

"I see letters falling, and I hear spinning carnival rides."

He thinks his mother can see and hear the daydreams too.

"You just have wild daydreams," she says.

"You know these stories are only imaginary."

"They aren't imaginary!" Daniel shouts. "They're real!"

Daniel's mother looks puzzled.

Axil chews on the letters.

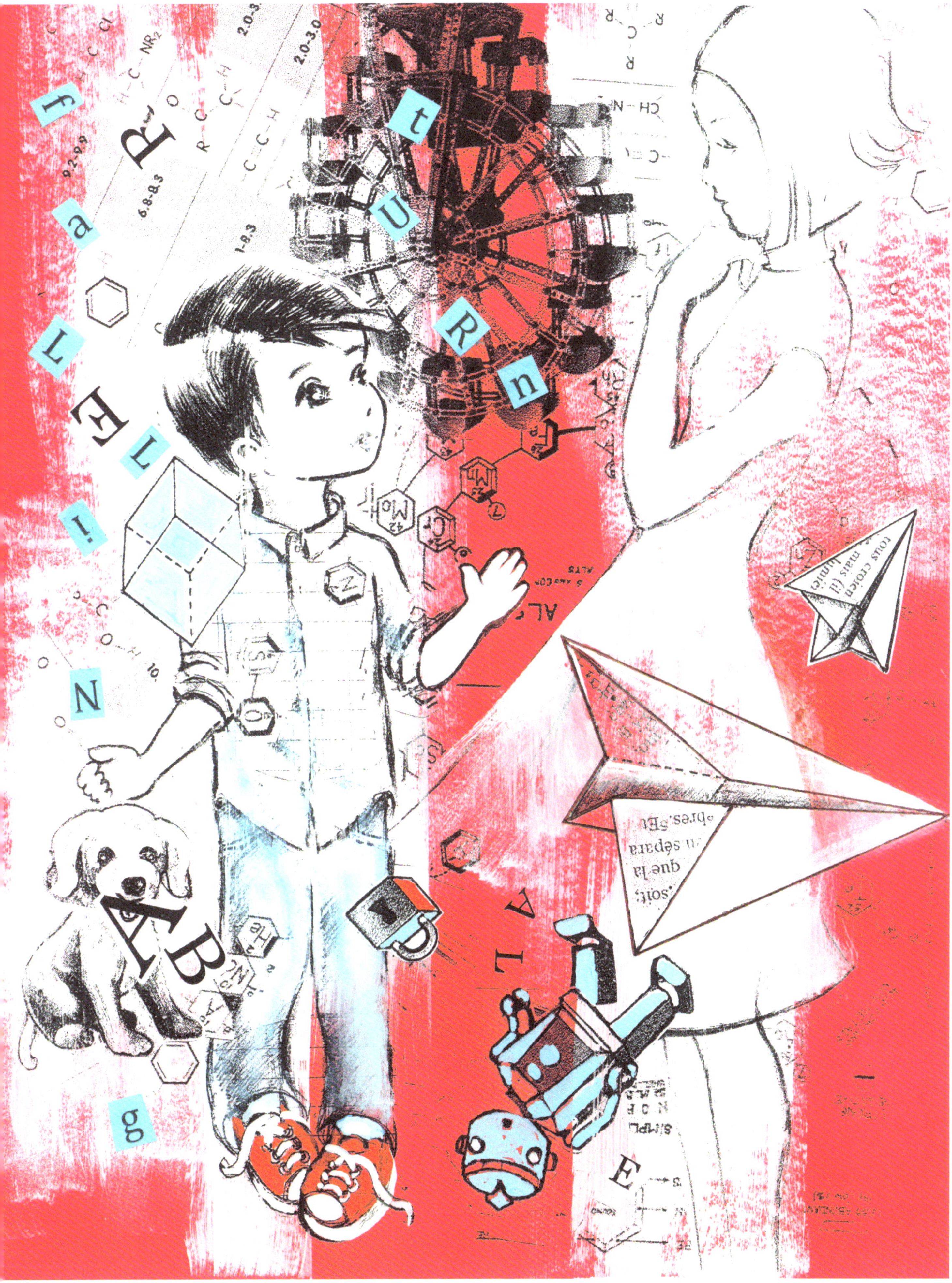

"My robot says he's real," Daniel says.

"Your robot isn't real," his mother replies.

"**Are *YOU* real?**" Daniel asks.

Daniel's mother takes the robot away.

"But ***all*** my toys tell me they're real!"

Axil says he's real, too.

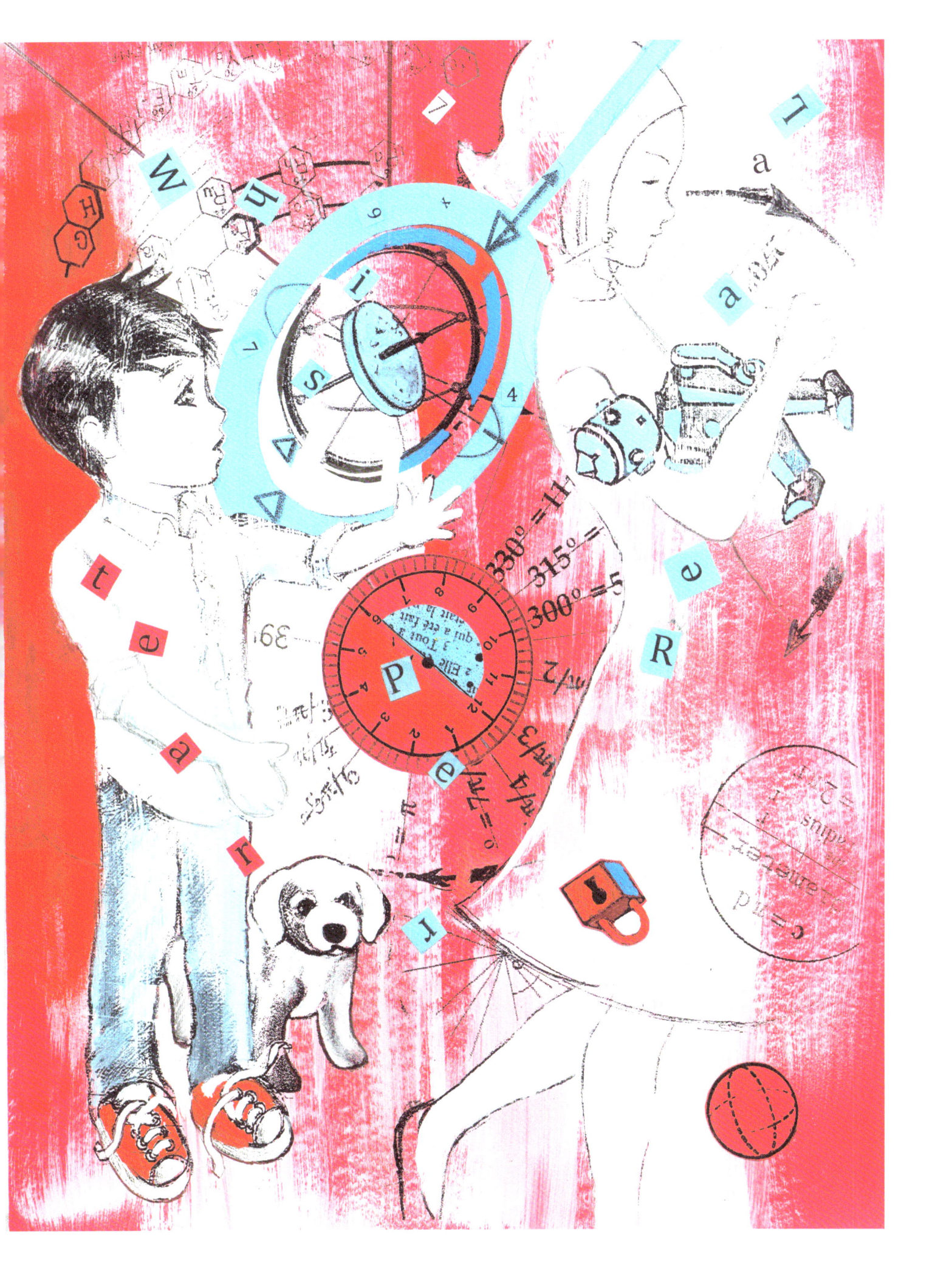

"They won't stop!" Daniel wails.

"What won't stop?"

"The voices!" Daniel answers. "And the daydreams!"

He sits on the floor.
He stares blankly at the wall.
Everything goes gray.

The voices stop.

"Daniel..." his mother whispers.
"Daniel?" she cries.

He doesn't blink.

"Daniel!" she anxiously waves her hand in front of his eyes.

He doesn't answer.

Axil barks.
Daniel doesn't even look at Axil.

Axil puts a paw on Daniel's arm.

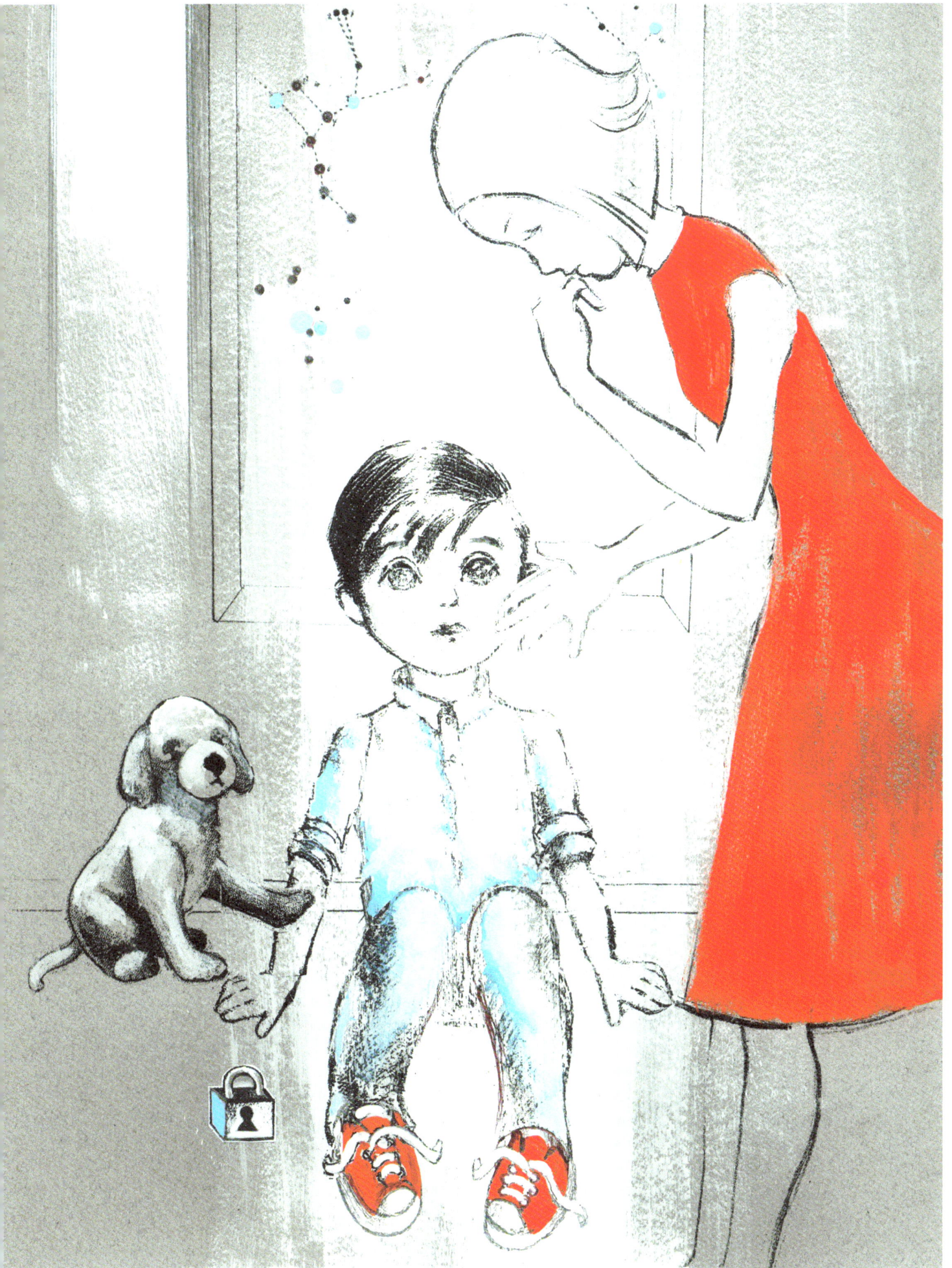

Daniel and his mother visit a psychiatrist, who helps care for
our minds and thoughts.

Axil has to stay home.

"Daniel, do you ever hear voices when nobody else is around?"
the psychiatrist asks.

"Yes."

"Do you ever see things that nobody else sees?"

"Yes."

"Do you ever believe things that don't seem real or true,

like a television is talking about you, or a toy is saying your thoughts?"

"Yes."

"How do these things make your thoughts feel?"

"Mixed up."

"How long has Daniel been talking about all this?" the psychiatrist asks.

"A long time," his mother replies.

Axil knows how long.

"Some of these things are real, Daniel, but some aren't," the psychiatrist
says. "They're symptoms of childhood schizophrenia, a thought disorder
that **mixes up our thoughts** about real things and daydreams. People with
schizophrenia have **hallucinations**; dreams you have when you're awake,
and **delusions**; thoughts you believe, that aren't true. Taking medicine helps
you ignore the "mixed-up" thoughts and focus on real things. When you begin
to take medicine, you might feel worse before you feel better. That only lasts a
few days. So don't give up!"

Axil never gives up.

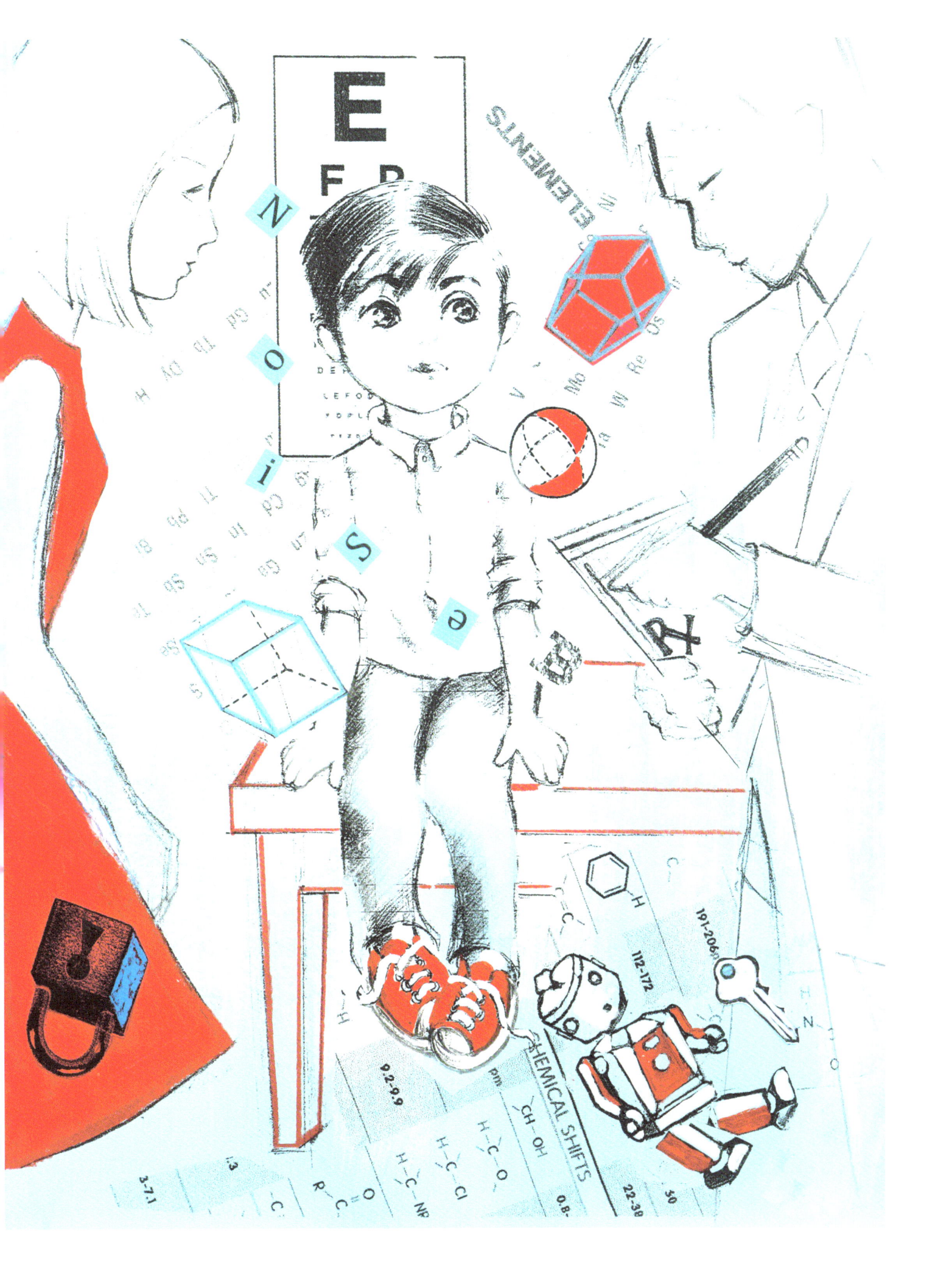

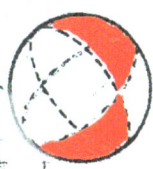

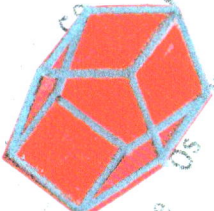

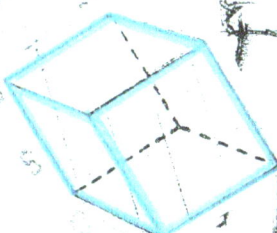

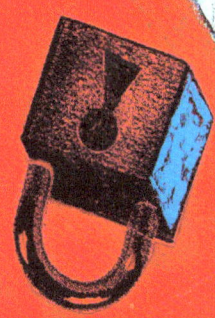

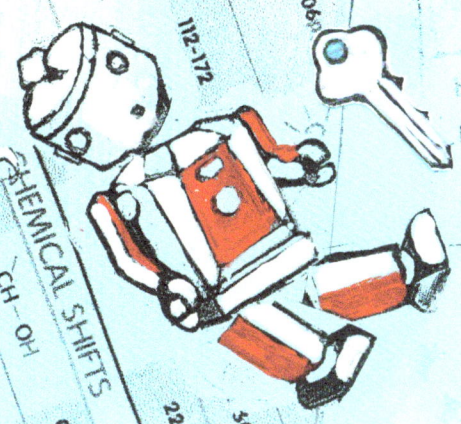

Next, Daniel and his mother visit a therapist, who helps us understand our emotions and feelings.

Axil has to stay home again.

"Can you draw a picture of how you feel?" the therapist asks.
Daniel draws himself with voices and objects in front of his face.

"What's going on in this picture?"

"Everything's noisy and crowded."

"How do these things make you feel?"

"Confused."

"What do you do when you feel confused?"

"I close my eyes, plug my ears, and wish it would all go away."

"Except for Axil."

"These are symptoms of childhood schizophrenia, Daniel, a thought disorder that makes us **feel confused** about real things and hallucinations", the therapist says. "Some kids call it crazy, but it's not. Just as kids with hearing or seeing disorders learn to hear or read differently, kids with thought disorders learn to control **confused feelings** differently. You can learn to focus *less* on feelings you ***don't*** want, and focus ***more*** on feelings you ***do*** want. When you learn to refocus and talk about all this, you might feel worse before you feel better. That won't last too long. So don't give up!"

Daniel draws Axil coloring in the lines.

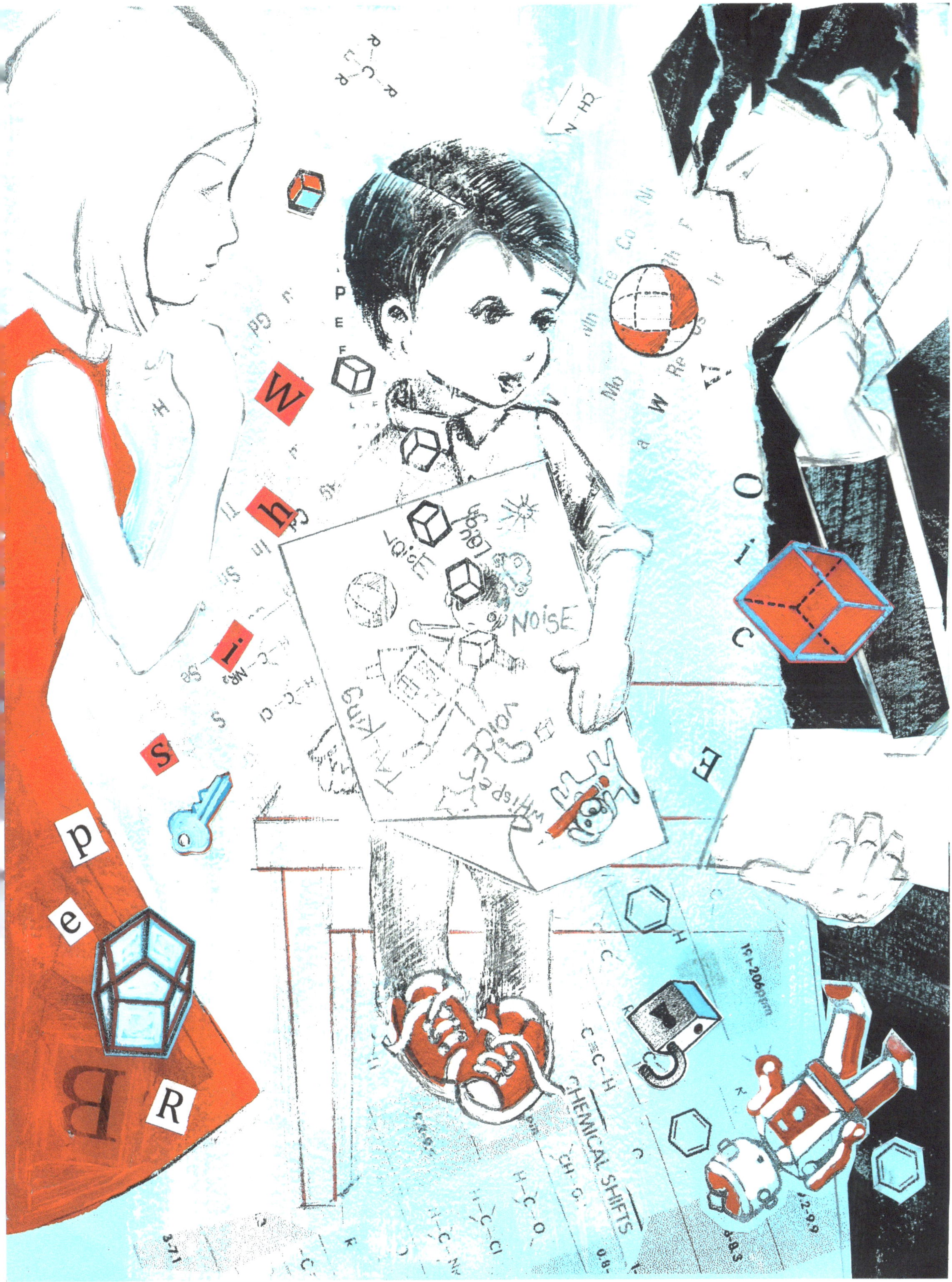
W
h
i
s
p
e
R
B
V
O
i
C
E
NOISE
CHEMICAL SHIFTS

Daniel starts taking medicine.

Some make him dizzy.
Some make him sleepy.
Some make him feel sick.

Daniel wants to give up.
But he remembers he might feel worse before he feels better.

After a few days, he stops feeling dizzy, sleepy and sick.
The medicine starts to work.
Many of the hallucinations and delusions begin to
fade away and quiet down.

He talks to the therapist and his mother about everything,
and they help him to know the difference between symptoms
and real things. Daniel begins to recognize
whether **some** things he sees, hears, feels and thinks are **real** or not.

At times all this talking makes him feel mixed up
and confused, and he wants to give up.
But he remembers that he might feel worse before he feels better.
And, he **does**.

Now he often feels calm and in control,
which he never felt before.

Daniel doesn't give up.

Axil doesn't either.

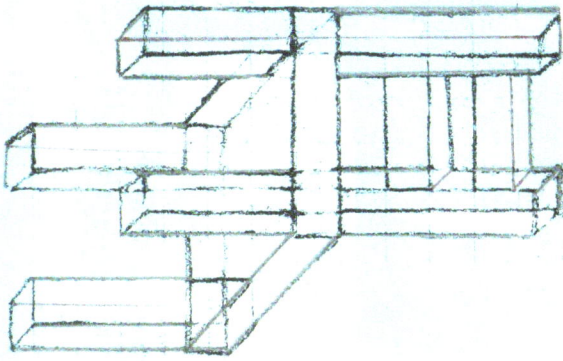
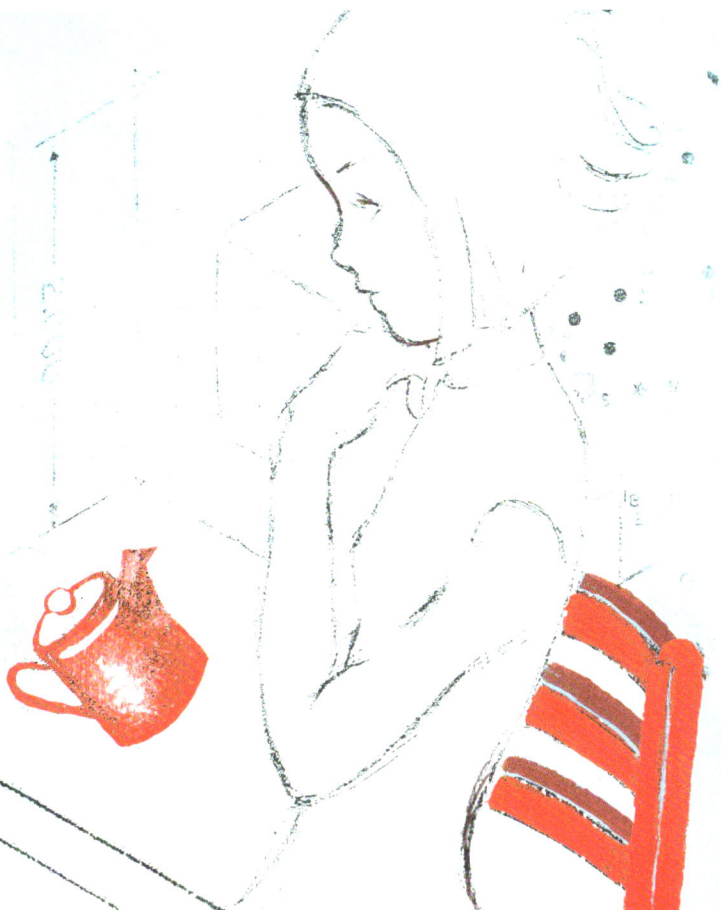
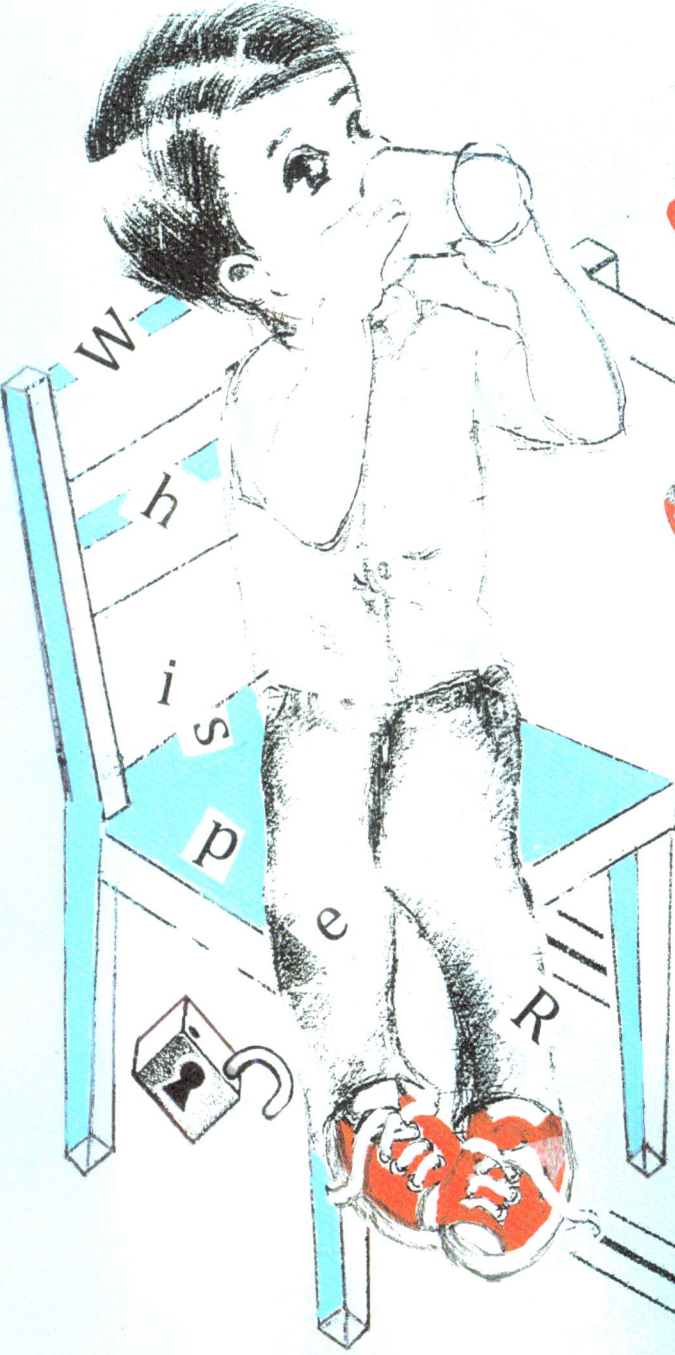
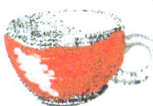
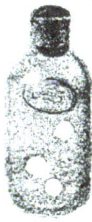
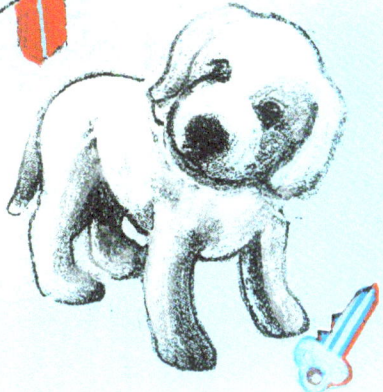

Daniel stops tripping over the daydreams.

Although, he still walks in a very slow and careful way.

He starts to make a friend.

Axil tugs the boy's shoelace.

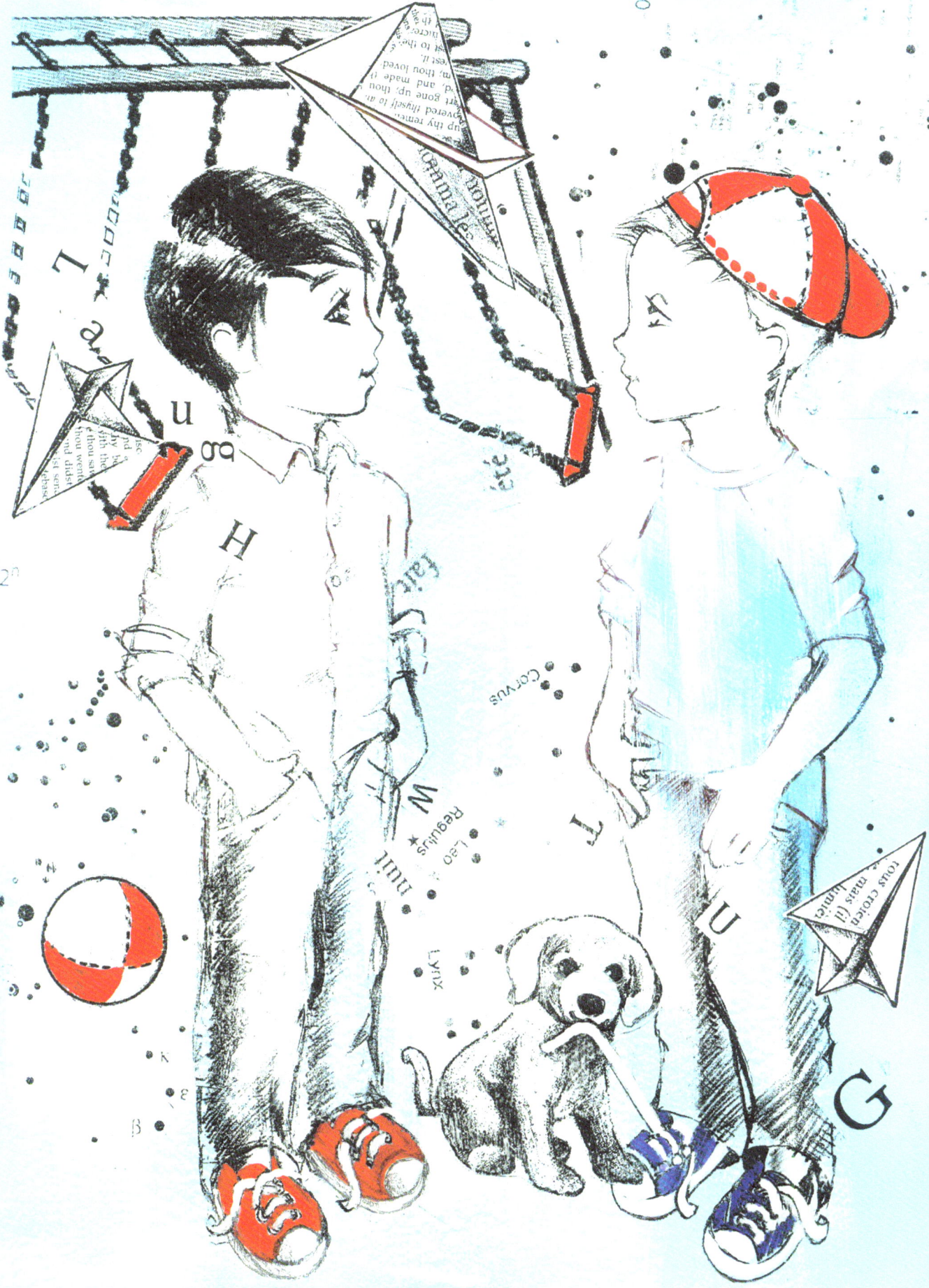

Daniel doesn't hear many loud voices anymore.

He's learning to ignore some of the daydreams.
Sometimes he can ignore them, but sometimes he can't.

Daniel knows now that **some** of the daydreams aren't real.

The daydreams used to be clear and loud.
Now they're often faded and quiet.

But the daydreams never really stop.

Although not everything's perfect in the daylight, it's okay.

Axil yawns, and sighs a big sigh.

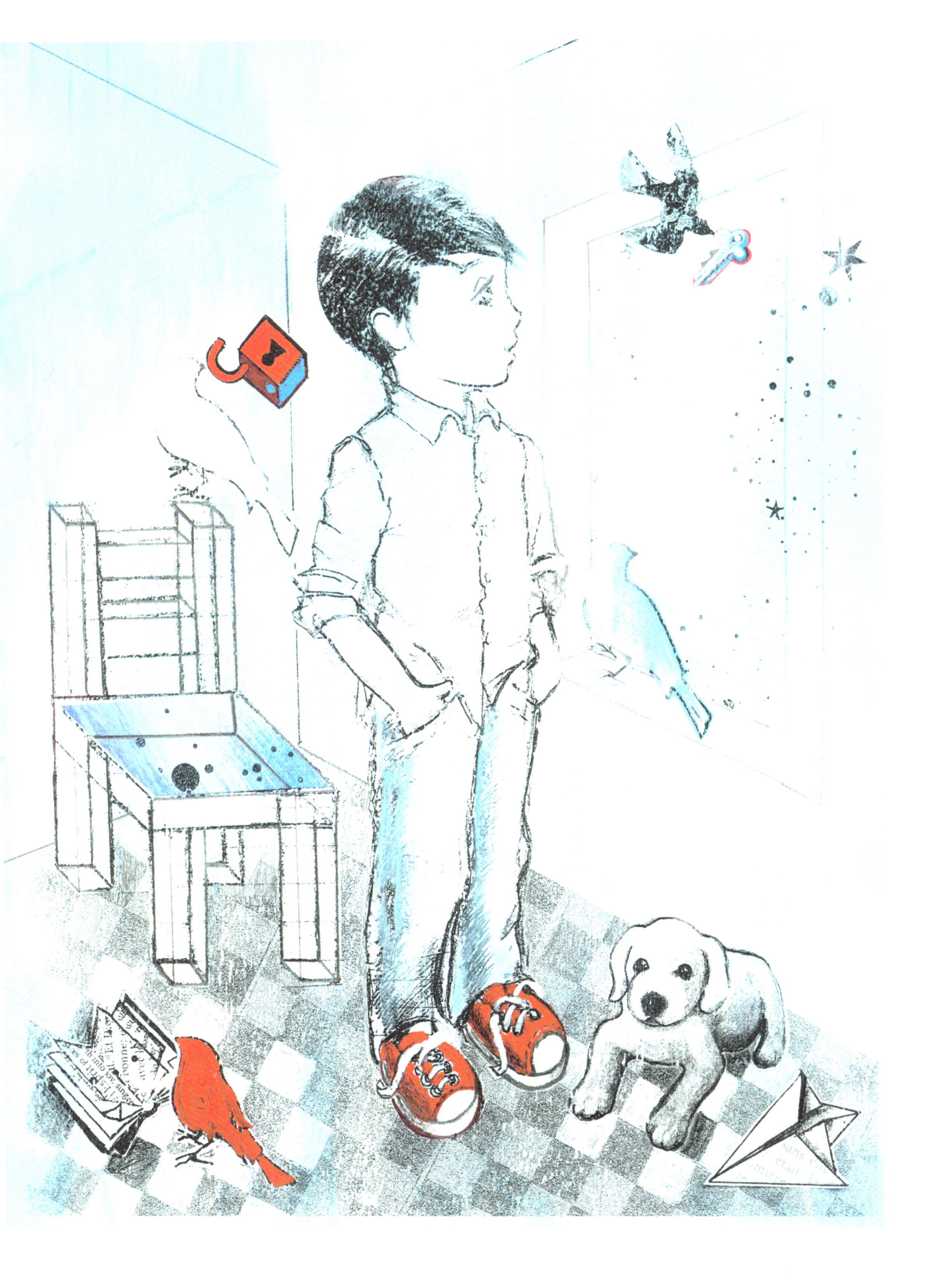

Daniel's night dreams don't seem so real any more.

And Axil doesn't mind sleeping with the lights off.

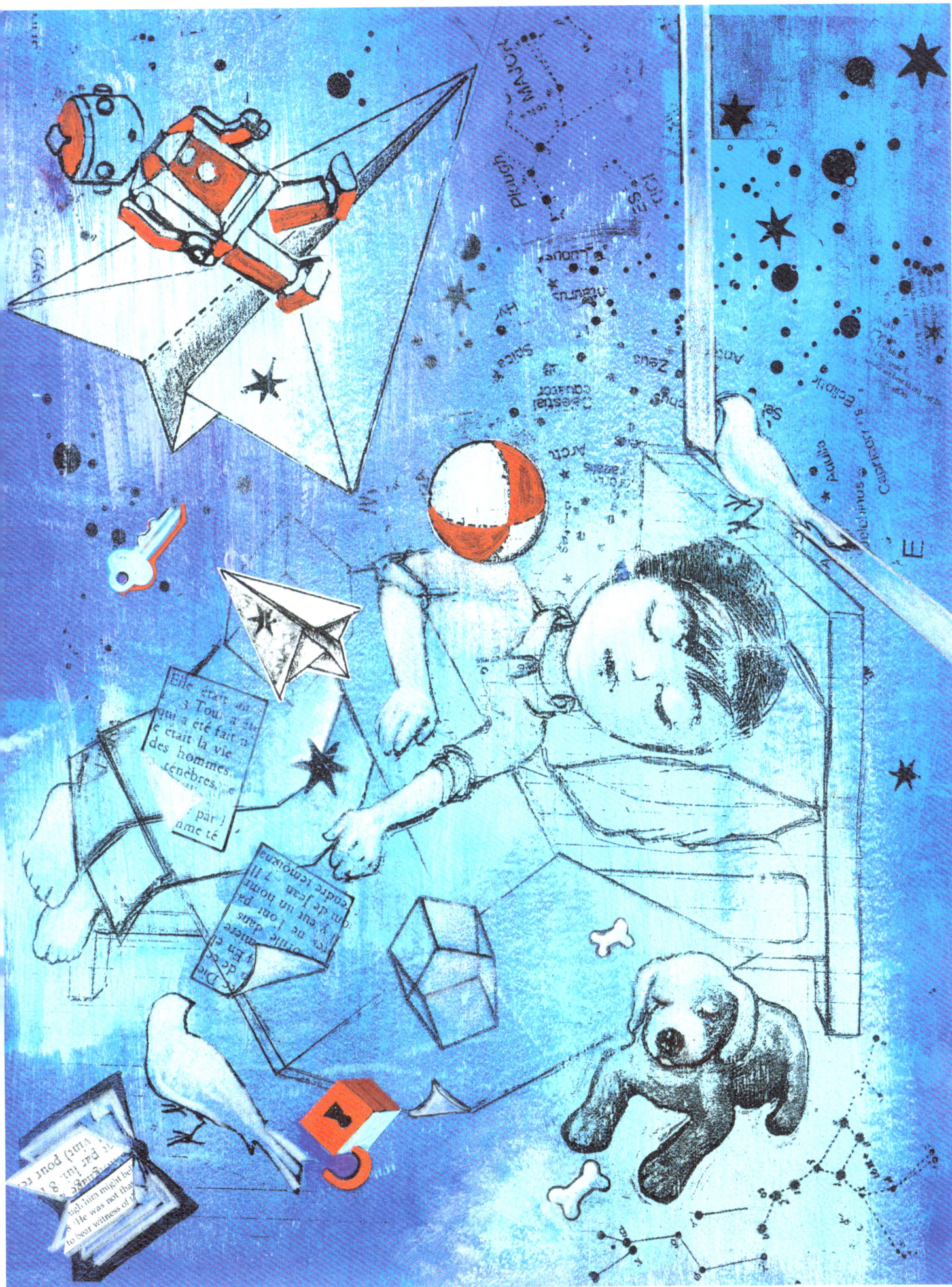

Acknowledgements

Thank you to my family for their understanding and support,
to Dr. Robert Byrnes and Dr. Todd Ivan for keeping me alive,
to William J. Miller and Dr. Jeffrey Morgan for staying by my
side as we were growing up while others thought I was odd
and remaining my friends until today, and to my co-author
and BFF Cynthia for being there for me in hard times
and good times.

— Daniel

Thank you to my children, Emma, Asher, and Clara,
to my sisters Kathy and Julie, to my parents, Ingrid
and Jozsi, and to my nieces Tahlia and Jenna, you are all
blessings to me. Thank you to Lydia, Giselle, Sabrina,
and their mother Evelyne, for whom my admiration grows
deeper each day. Thank you to Daniel, an inspiration
and a true friend. Lastly, thank you to my husband Kyle,
about whom Dr. Seuss perfectly described,
 "...I meant what I said and I said what I meant,
an elephant's faithful one hundred percent."

— Cynthia

About the Authors

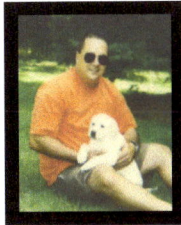

Daniel-James F. Clarke, whose childhood this book memoirs, has an MA in counseling psychology and has been an adjunct math professor at a state college. He is a US Army veteran, and has a son, Ryan-Christopher, in the US Army who recently returned from Afghanistan. Daniel raised his son as a single father while battling schizophrenia, bipolar disorder, anxiety disorder and PTSD. He loves dogs.

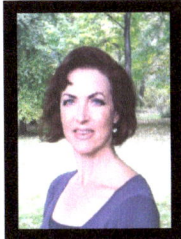

Cynthia Kaufman Rose, MFA, is an exhibiting professional artist. She has been an adjunct art professor at several colleges, an Ohio Arts Council artist in residence in primary and secondary schools, and was awarded several Ohio Arts Council artist fellowships. Having bipolar disorder opened a door to transform her poetic imagery and words into a voice advocating for children. She is married to Kyle, and they have three children, Emma, Asher and Clara.

www.ingramcontent.com/pod-product-compliance
Lightning Source LLC
Chambersburg PA
CBHW060825270326

41931CB00002B/65